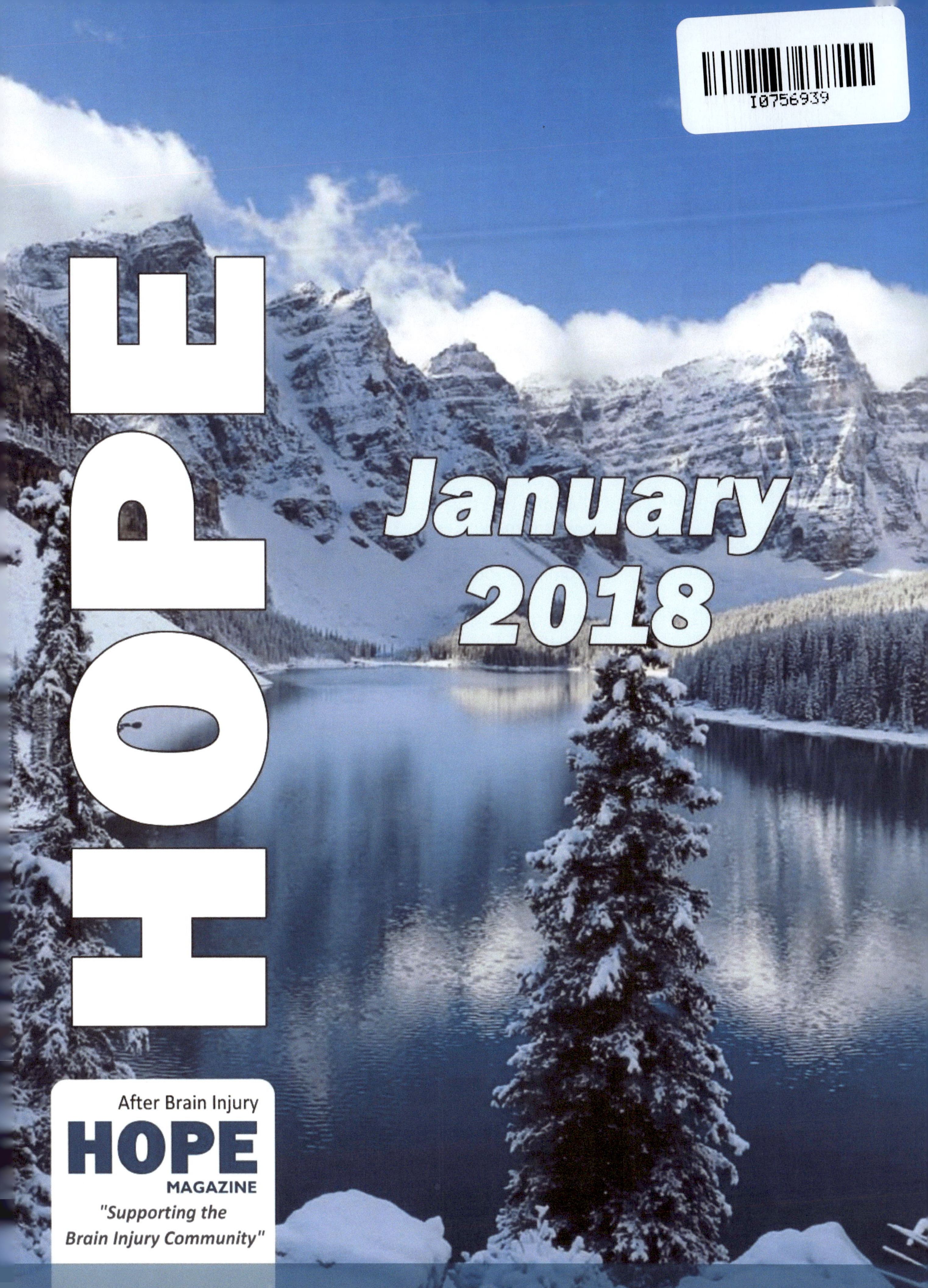

HOPE
January
2018
After Brain Injury
HOPE
MAGAZINE
"Supporting the
Brain Injury Community"
I0756939

Welcome

HOPE MAGAZINE

Serving All Impacted by Brain Injury

January 2018

Publisher
David A. Grant

Editor
Sarah Grant

Contributing Writers
Stacia Bissell
Jen Dodge
Donna O'Donnell Figurski
David A. Grant
Paul McMonagle
Ted Stachulski
Carole Starr
Barbara Webster

Amazing Cartoonist
Patrick Brigham

FREE subscriptions at
www.TBIHopeMagazine.com

Welcome to the January 2018 issue of HOPE Magazine!

January is a time for new beginnings, a time for reflection, and for many, a time to make changes.

We are pleased to ring in the new year more focused than ever on serving those with lives that have been touched by brain injury. A recent survey of our social community showed that our community is indeed a mix of all types of brain injury, both traumatic and otherwise.

Mindful that this has been the trend for a couple of years now, we are making some exciting changes here to better serve the brain injury community. You can read more about what is coming in our first story, Hope After Brain Injury.

A warm "welcome back!" to our regular readers. For those new to HOPE Magazine, our New Year's wish is that you find something here that helps you along your own personal journey.

Peace,

David A. Grant
Publisher

Contents

What's Inside

January 2018

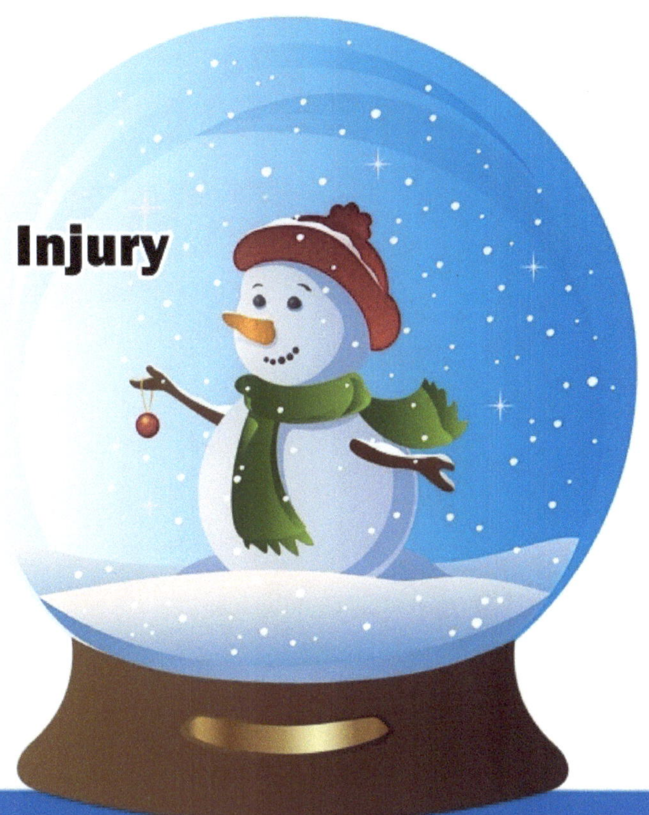

"Write it on your heart that every day is the best day in the year."

~Ralph Waldo Emerson

HOPE MAGAZINE

Volume Discount Program

With our volume pricing program, your qualifying organization can purchase print copies of HOPE Magazine for up to 50% off!

Perfect for...

Brain Injury Support Groups

Area Agencies & Case Workers

Healthcare Professionals

Brain Injury Associations

Brain Injury Alliances

Call 603-898-4540 to Learn More!

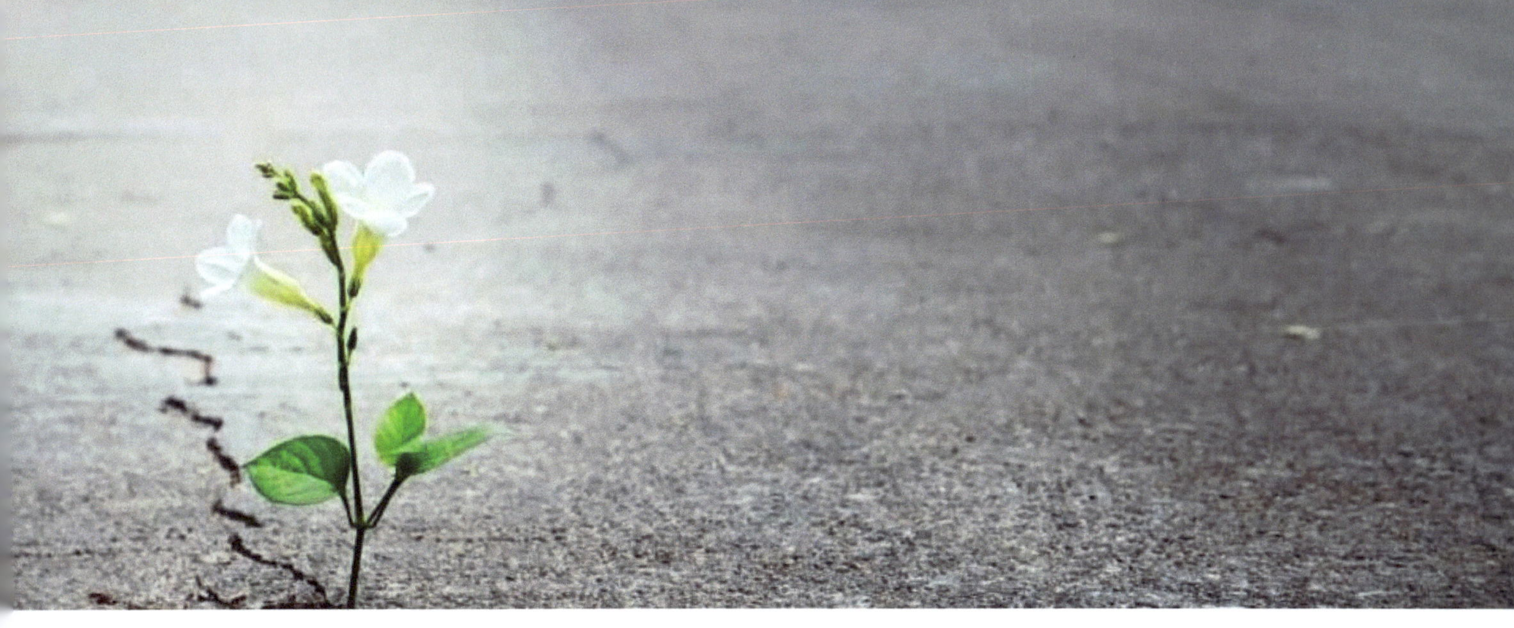

HOPE After Brain Injury
By David A. Grant

We are in the midst of some sweeping changes in both our publication as well as our website. But before we look forward, let's look back, back to a late fall day in 2010.

It all started innocently enough. A middle-aged guy went out for his daily bike ride, but the day ended far from innocently. I was "that guy," the person t-boned by a newly licensed driver. The date was November 11, 2010. Like so many other brain injury survivors, I often measure my life in two parts, the before and the after.

Life "before" my injury was pretty average. I was newly married to the girl of my dreams. We had a bright and promising future. Self-employed at the time, my web design business was thriving, the kids were healthy, and the mortgage was always paid on time. We had a simple, uneventful life.

What could possibly go wrong?

> "Brain injury does have a way of shaking up life a bit."

The "after" has unfolded in a way neither my wife Sarah nor I ever could have foreseen. Brain injury does have a way of shaking up life a bit. During my first post-injury year, I began attending a local face-to-face support group. Once a month, I was in the presence of those who "get it" about brain injury. But for twenty-nine days between our meetings, we all flew solo again, no longer in the company of our peers.

We started a small Facebook group - a group that allowed us all to stay in touch with each other between our regular meetings. Though that first Facebook group doesn't see much activity these days, it served its purpose. Something amazing happens when survivors are together. There is a healing in peer-to-peer support that you can find nowhere else.

Back in 2013, as I began a new journey as a brain injury advocate, I began to hear story after story of survivors who were isolated, either by geography, or by physical post-injury limitations. When I founded the TBI HOPE and Inspiration Facebook community, I envisioned a smaller group, a safe place where folks from anywhere could stop by, spend a bit of time in the presence of peers, and move on in their respective days.

Suffice to say, things did not go the way I had initially envisioned.

Today, our Facebook community is one of the world's largest social communities focused solely on brain injury. With tens of thousands of members, we come together from over forty countries and all walks of life. It has become one of the most amazing experiences that I have ever been part of – and one you just cannot see coming.

With the passage of time, as Sarah and I continued to serve others, we continued to learn more about the brain injury community. One of the most surprising lessons learned was that many of the members of the TBI Hope and Inspiration community did not have traumatic brain injuries. In my early naiveté, I thought that every brain injury was traumatic. What can I say? I am a layperson who learns as he goes, and not a member of the medical community.

Over the years, the TBI HOPE and Inspiration community grew to include thousands of members who had non-traumatic injuries. Stroke survivors found a home and comfort in the presence of others. So did those with anoxic brain injury. Family members and caregivers now make up a large percentage of our group's membership.

However, I continued to be plagued by a lingering uneasiness. Though welcomed, some members still felt out of place, with several reaching out to me directly asking if it was okay to be part of the group without a traumatic brain injury.

Last year, Sarah and I charted the next chapter of our organization. We developed a mission statement.

"Our Mission is to Advocate, Educate, and Serve all Affected by Brain Injury."

Mindful of our mission to serve ALL affected by brain injury, we now are in the midst of making some sweeping changes that will allow people with all types of brain injury to feel welcome. We are now moving forward with our new name, *Hope After Brain Injury*. This seemingly small name change has gigantic implications. There is now no limiting qualifier that may lead some to question whether they belong and are welcome in our community.

Some of the changes are already in place. Before my injury, I was a professional web developer by trade. As my own recovery continued to progress, I was able to return to work in a profession that I love. Last year was the first year that I jumped back into web design work after a six-year hiatus. So much for that old theory that recovery ends in a year.

In December, we rolled out the all-new *Hope After Brain Injury* website. Gone is most of the limiting verbiage about traumatic brain injury. With the re-launch of our site comes a new focus. Our vision for the new site is one of being an information and support destination for all affected by brain injury.

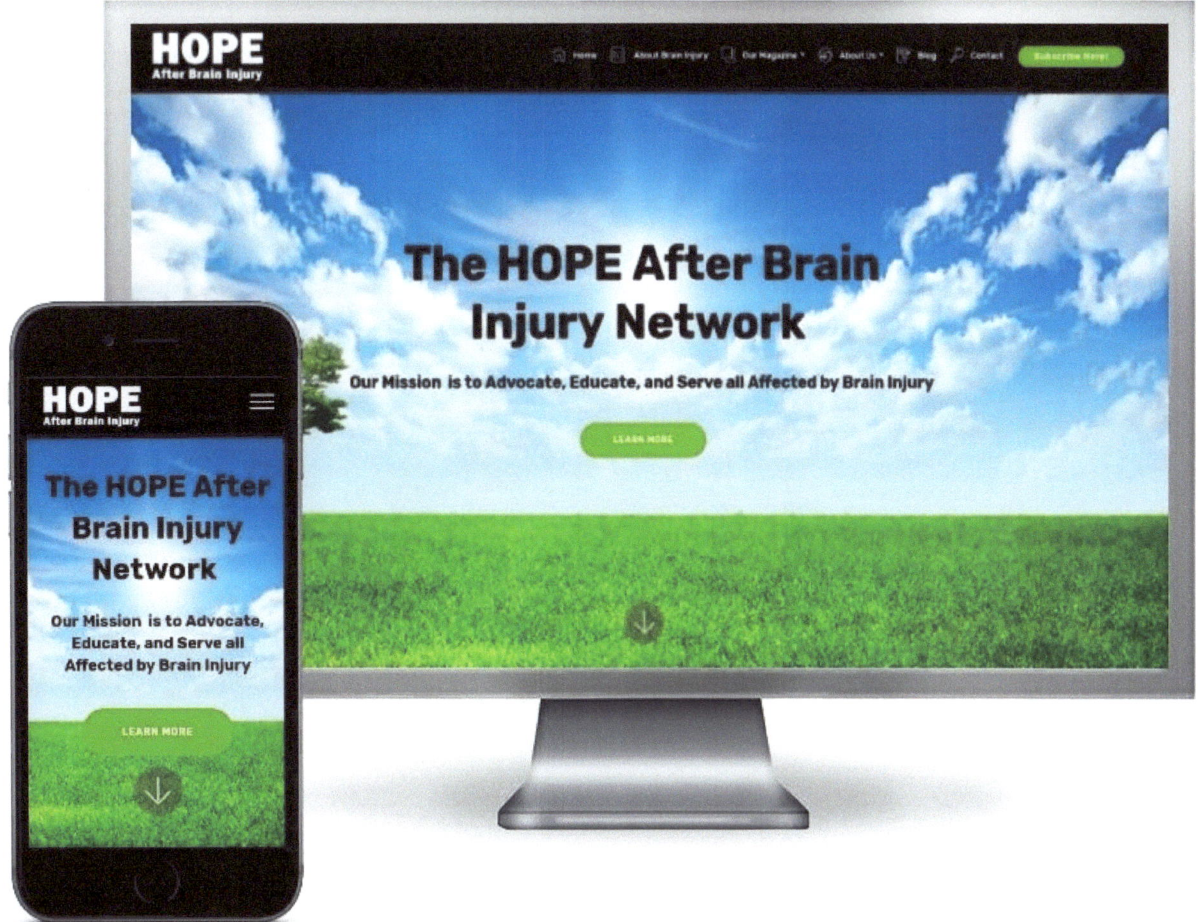

We already have a state-by-state nationwide directory of every Brain Injury Association and Alliance. Over the months that come, we will be adding many more additional local resources, making the *Hope After Brain Injury* website the most robust single-source of meaningful information worldwide. If this sounds like a lofty goal, it's because it is. Our record of accomplishment has given us the confidence that we really can do almost anything.

As we grow the site content through 2018, we will be adding a very robust personal stories section where first-time and regular site visitors can find common ground with others living lives after brain injury. Many will find the end of isolation in the words of others.

Our new site is built using an entirely different architecture than the legacy website. Built using next-generation responsive design, mobile users will have the same great experience as desktop users have. I hold the development of our new site very close to my heart. At a year post-injury, I was told by a well-respected member of the medical community that my recovery was over. Having the ability to both learn and implement a new type of web development has been exhilarating for me personally. For a few years, I thought my life was over. Time has shown that it is not. Other social presences like our Twitter page, Pinterest Page, and YouTube video channel will retain the same addresses, though the forward-facing graphics will change to better reflect our new name.

In this same spirit, our monthly magazine will now be published under a simple and straightforward name. Our January 2018 issue is the first issue with our new name - HOPE Magazine. It will continue to serve the brain injury community as it has done for almost three years.

If it sounds as if we have a lot on our plates, we do. There are millions of brain injuries annually worldwide, yet a void in meaningful, forward-moving, and healing information still exists. If we can fill even a small piece of that void, lives will be made easier and humanity will be lifted higher.

This is not a solo endeavor. I welcome your thoughts and input. If you've got an idea about how we can better serve those who need it most, I'd love to hear from you. To those who have found a safe haven in the HOPE community, it is because of you that we've all come this far.

Meet David A. Grant

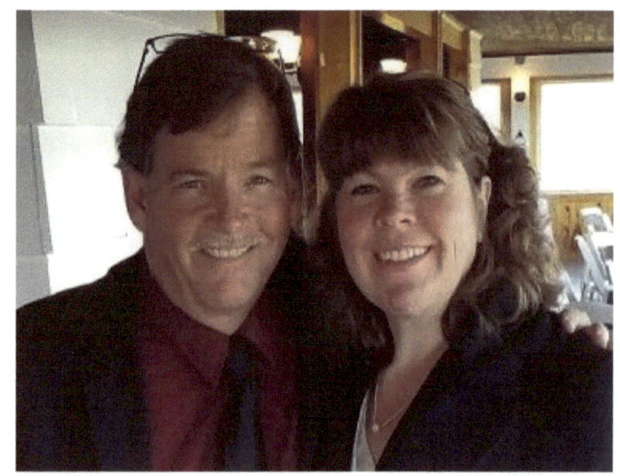

David A. Grant is a freelance writer based out of southern New Hampshire and the publisher of HOPE Magazine. He is the author of Metamorphosis, Surviving Brain Injury.

He is also a contributing author to Chicken Soup for the Soul, Recovering from Traumatic Brain Injuries. David is a BIANH Board Member as well as a regular contributing writer to Brainline.org, a PBS sponsored website.

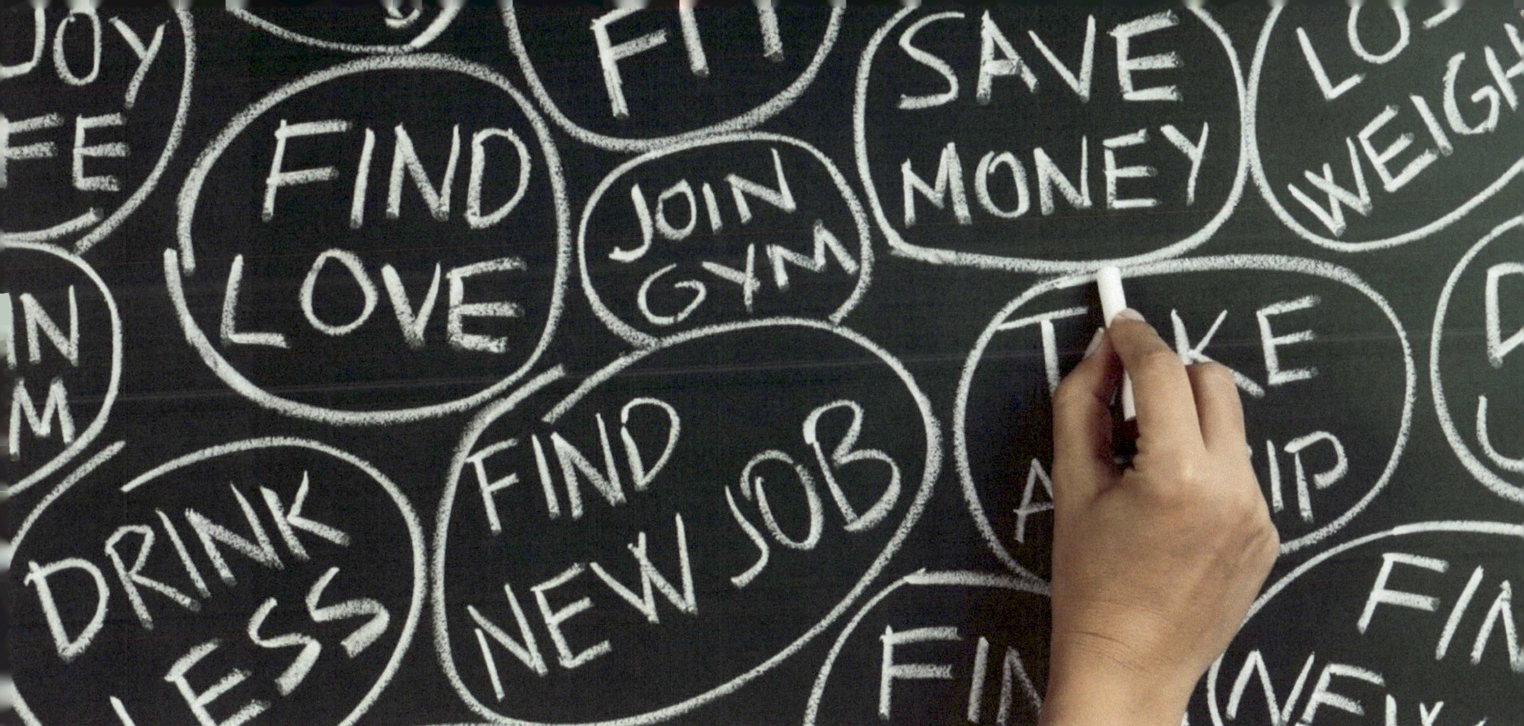

Resolutions for Brain Injury Survivors

By Carole Starr

After brain injury, it's common to look at the past and grieve who we used to be. There's so much loss to process, it may seem impossible to face a future with a brain that doesn't work the same anymore. There are mindsets that can support us while we work on gradually accepting our new selves.

When you resolve to incorporate new ways of thinking into your life, you can begin to transition from looking backward at the past to facing forward toward the future. You can begin to move from surviving to thriving after brain injury.

Resolutions are something most of us associate with a new year. Some scholars say that the month of January was named for the ancient Roman god Janus. Janus had two faces looking in opposite directions. One stared backward toward the past, while the other gazed forward toward the future. Because Janus simultaneously looked at the past and future, he symbolized beginnings and endings and transition spaces like doorways and bridges.

> **You can begin to move from surviving to thriving after brain injury.**

Janus is the perfect symbol for the New Year, when many people take the time to reflect on their lives over the previous twelve months and to plan ahead for the next twelve.

Janus can also be a symbol for the brain injury acceptance process. Whatever the date of your brain injury, that day becomes a metaphorical January 1st. It's the date that sharply divides your life into two halves. Our language reflects that divide. We talk about our old self versus our new self and our old life versus our new life. Every moment in life is categorized as happening either before the brain injury or after the brain injury.

Acceptance can be defined as being like Janus and looking at both the past and the future. When we've accepted brain injury, we're able to acknowledge the past without getting overwhelmed by emotion. At the same time, we're able to face the future and live within a new normal.

I spent many years after my brain injury looking backward at the life and the self I lost. I mourned deeply who I'd been and the promise that seemed to be gone. A future living with my brain injury deficits seemed much too scary and depressing to even consider. It took me about eight years to work through that heavy grief and to transition to facing forward into acceptance of my new life as a brain injury survivor.

If you're someone who feels stuck right now looking back at the past, you may be wondering something like this: 'But how can I transition from looking backward to looking forward?' One thing I learned in my own brain injury journey was that how I thought about my experience mattered. I couldn't control the brain injury, but I did have some control over how I thought about it. There were some mindsets that kept me trapped in all the loss and others that facilitated my movement forward. Our thoughts can have great power.

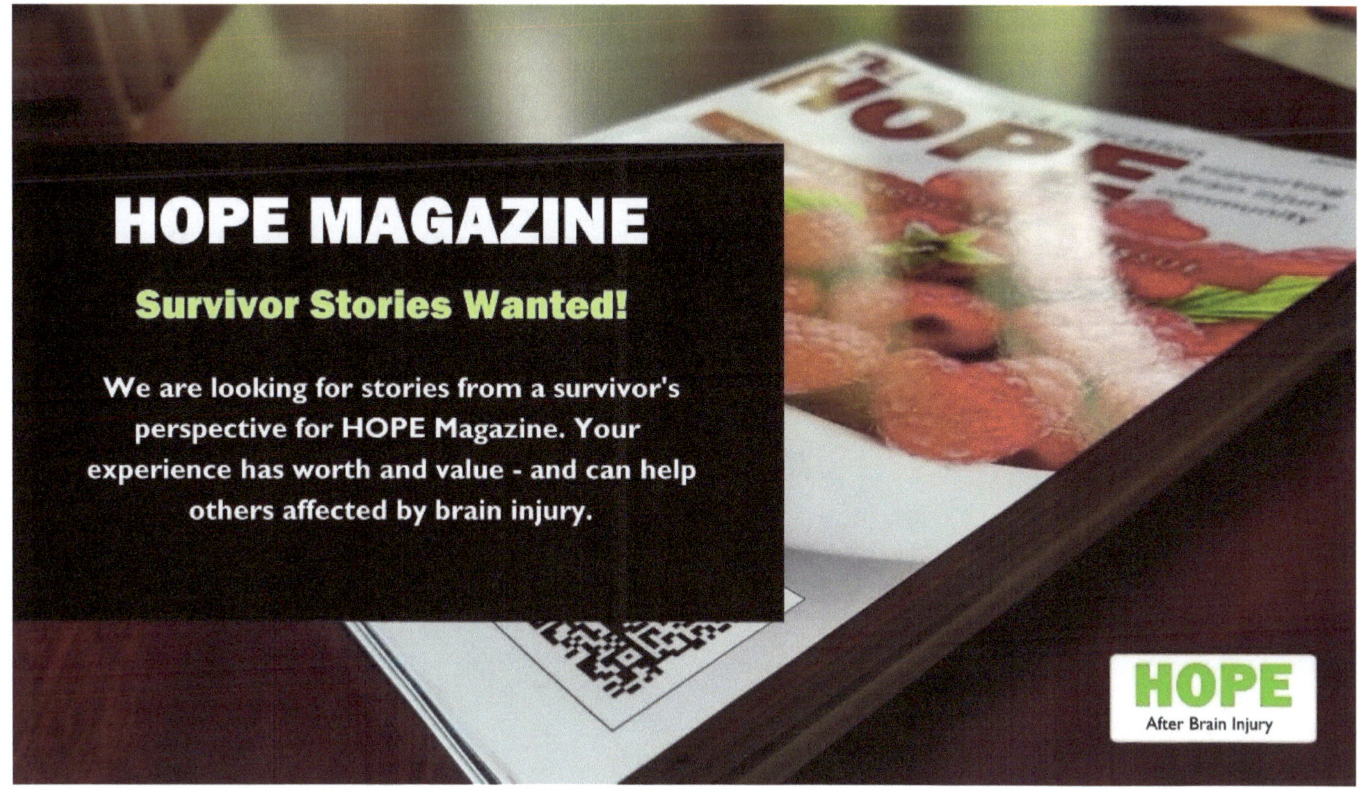

Here are five mindsets that helped me in my journey to acceptance. I hope they are helpful in yours too. I have worded these mindsets as resolutions, because that turns them into items for action. Acceptance is an action-oriented process. It's with resolve that we can turn toward the future.

These resolutions will not be accomplished overnight or even all at once. They require time, patience and persistence. As you read the resolutions, note which one or ones stand out for you. That will give you clues where you are ready to grow and begin to face forward.

Resolutions for Brain Injury Survivors

I Resolve to Recognize and Celebrate my Progress
No matter how slow and uneven the progress happens or how small and inconsequential the gains may seem, I will savor every step forward. My successes will build on one another.

I Resolve to Stop Comparing
It's not fair to compare my new self to who I used to be or to compare my brain injury to others' brain injuries. Both types of comparison only set me up for extra grief and feeling inferior. Instead, I'll use the day of my brain injury as my starting point. It will be my personal New Year's and I'll measure my progress from there. My journey is my own and will not match anyone else's.

I Resolve to be Gentle with Myself when I Fail
I'm doing my best. Every failure gives me an opportunity to learn and grow.

I Resolve to Find an Activity that my Current Self is Good at and Can Enjoy
The more I focus on what I can do, the better I'll feel about myself.

I Resolve to Trust that my Life can Still be Good
Where I am right now in my journey isn't where I'll always be. I'll continue to grow, to change and to learn. My life may never be the same again, but it doesn't have to be ruined.

When I was working on incorporating these resolutions into my life, I had copies of them strategically placed in various locations around my house. That way I had to read them multiple times a day. This helped them gradually seep into my way of thinking. I even framed some of them and hung them on my wall.

The resolutions were also the topic of many conversations with my family, friends, brain injury support group and various medical professionals. They gently encouraged me when my thoughts were stuck and all I could see was everything I'd lost to brain injury.

Resolutions like these can help us move from looking backward at the past to looking forward to the future. I encourage you to think about ways to incorporate them into your own life.

Meet Carole Starr

Carole Starr sustained a brain injury in a car accident in 1999. She was unable to return to her career as a teacher or to her hobby of classical musical performance. Carole has reinvented herself by focusing on what she can do, one small step at a time. She's now an inspiring keynote speaker and the leader of Brain Injury Voices, an award-winning survivor education, advocacy and peer mentoring group in Maine.

Carole's newest role is that of author. This selection is an excerpt from her recently published book, To Root & To Rise: Accepting Brain Injury. To learn more about Carole, her speeches and her book, please visit CaroleJStarr.com

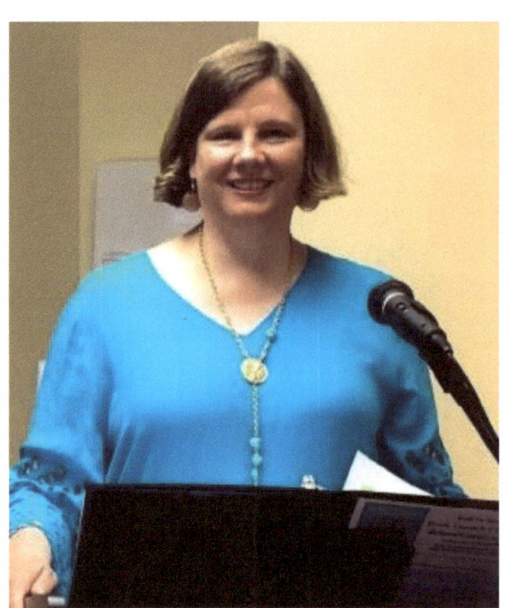

Everything passes, but nothing entirely goes away.

~Jenny Diski

All concussions are serious.
If you think you have a

CONCUSSION:

* Don't hide it.
* Report it.
* Take time to recover.

HEADACHE

PRESSURE IN HEAD

NAUSEA OR VOMITING

BALANCE PROBLEMS
OR DIZZINESS

DOUBLE OR
BLURRY VISION

SENSITIVITY TO
LIGHT OR NOISE

FEELING SLUGGISH, HAZY,
FOGGY, OR GROGGY

CONCENTRATION OR
MEMORY PROBLEMS

CONFUSION

JUST NOT "FEELING RIGHT"
OR "FEELING DOWN"

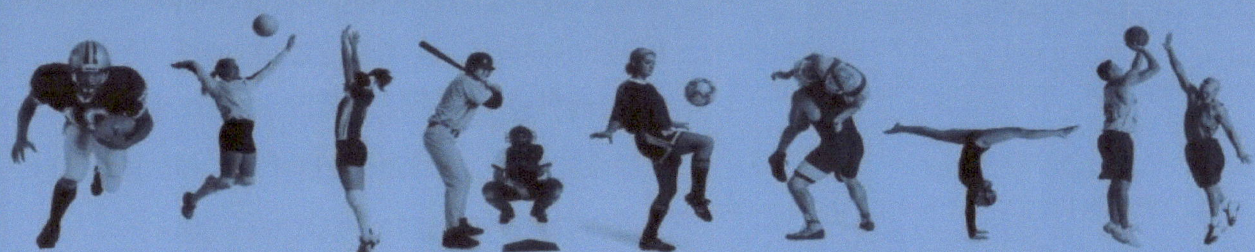

It's better to miss one game than the whole season.

For more information and to order additional materials *free-of-charge*, visit: www.cdc.gov/Concussion.

U.S. DEPARTMENT OF HEALTH AND HUMAN SERVICES
CENTERS FOR DISEASE CONTROL AND PREVENTION

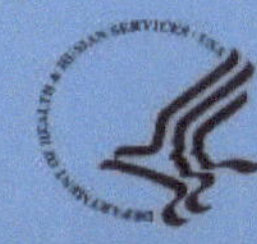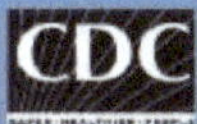

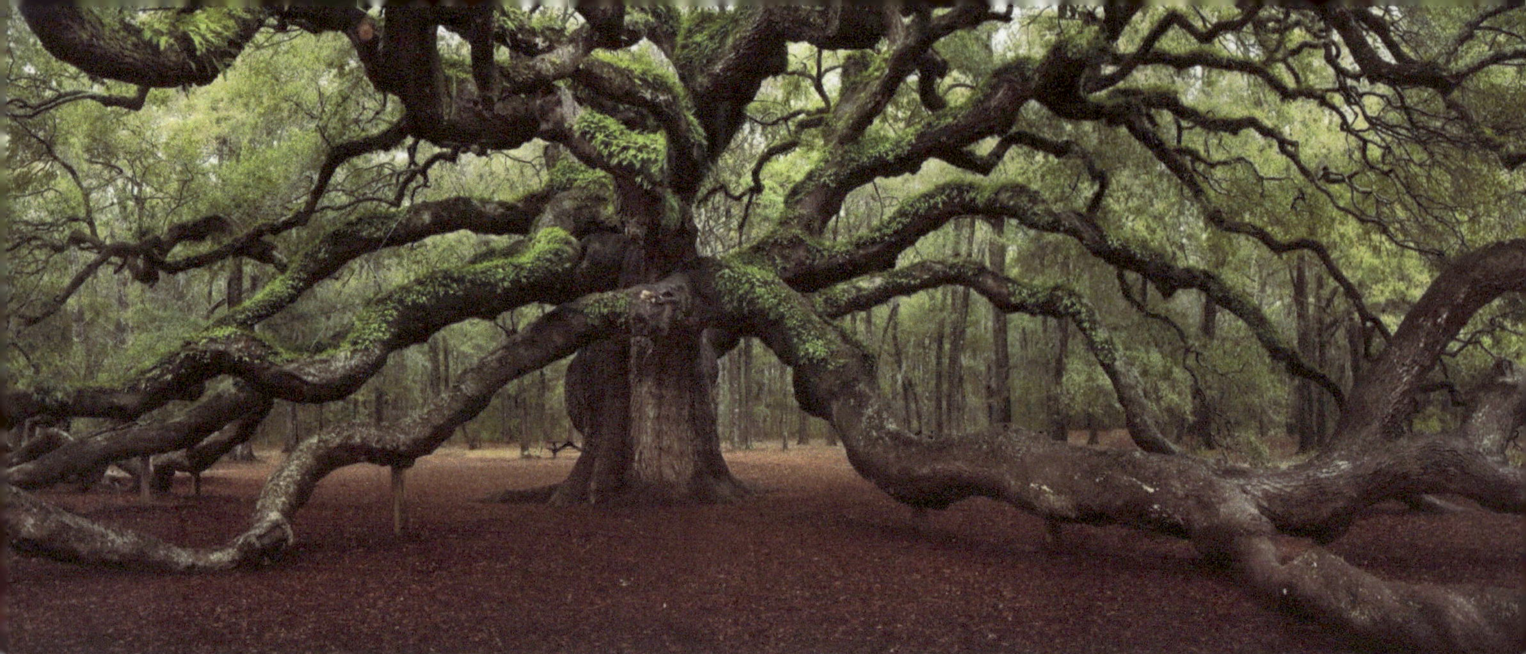

Angel Oak
By Barbara Webster

Angel Oak grows majestically in a small peaceful park on Johns Island, near Charleston, South Carolina. This legendary tree is a southern live oak tree over 66 feet tall and 28 feet around, with limbs that spread over 187 feet. It is estimated to be over 400 years old! Imagine that! Imagine what it could tell us about the past 400 years? Imagine what its advice would be to us?

While on vacation several years ago, as I stood in wonder under its enormous canopy, my thoughts drifted to the far-reaching, long lasting, effects of brain injury. At the time, I was involved in a poetry project with brain injury survivors. Our writings echoed the far-reaching, long lasting, painful difficulties and complex challenges of being a brain injury survivor.

> **Our writings echoed the far-reaching, long lasting, painful difficulties and complex challenges of being a brain injury survivor.**

When I saw this phenomenal tree, with its widespread branches and countless leaves, I knew it was perfect for the cover of my project. If you look closely, you will notice that the branches are not straight but bend and curve in different directions. Some are even propped up. Angel Oak was damaged severely during Hurricane Hugo in 1989 - but it is thriving!

Recently, as I was browsing the local card store, I was drawn to a card with a picture of a tree. It looked familiar. . . When I moved closer, I was delighted to discover that the picture of the tree on the card was the same tree that had inspired me years before. As I read the accompanying poem, it spoke to me and touched my heart, just like the poems of the brain injury survivors in that poetry project years ago; with an understanding and wisdom that only someone who has experienced a critical life event like a brain injury would be able to express.

I knew I had to share it with my fellow brain injury survivors. I hope it will resonate with you as profoundly as it does with me, validating your strength and courage and giving you Hope.

The Oak Tree

A mighty wind blew night and day.
It stole the oak tree's leaves away,
Then snapped its boughs and pulled its bark
Until the oak was tired and stark.
But still the oak tree held its ground
While other trees fell all around.

The weary wind gave up and spoke,
"How can you still be standing, Oak?"
The oak tree said, "I know that you
Can break each branch of mine in two,
Carry every leaf away,
Shake my limbs, and make me sway.
But I have roots stretched in the earth,
Growing stronger since my birth.

You'll never touch them, for you see,
They are the deepest part of me.
Until today, I wasn't sure
Of just how much I could endure.
But now I've found, with thanks to you,
I'm stronger than I ever knew."

~Johnny Ray Ryder Jr.

Meet Barbara Webster

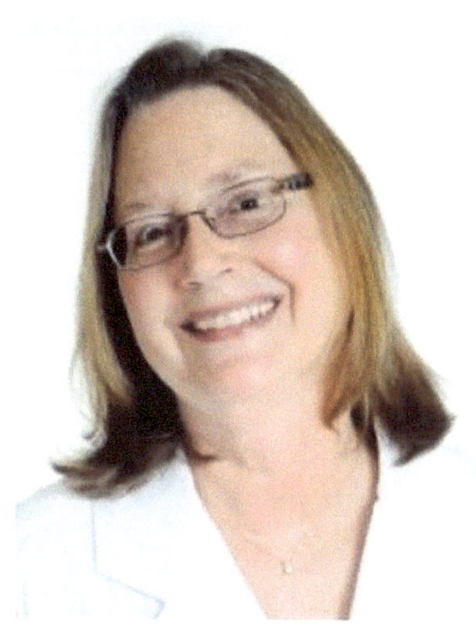

Barbara J. Webster is the author of "Lost and Found, A Survivor's Guide for Reconstructing Life after Brain Injury." She is also a contributor to "Chicken Soup for the Traumatic Brain Injury Survivor's Soul." Barbara works for the Brain Injury Association of MA as the Survivor & Caregiver Educator.

Several excerpts from her book, including the popular "What Brain Injury Survivors Want You to Know" and the PhotoVoice Projects from the Amazing Brain Injury Survivor Support Group in Framingham, MA can be found on Brainline.org.

The Harsh Reality

By Jen Dodge

Approximately two years ago, I needed to change my work schedule. I began working fewer hours in an attempt to help my rattled brain heal. It did not take long for the comments to start. Comments such as, "It must be nice not working full-time," or "I wish I was you." Trust me on this one, you do not want to wish you were me. For me, working fewer hours (or not working at all) is not a vacation.

I partially blame myself for people's lack of understanding. Like many others, I hide what I am going through a lot. When I cannot disguise it, I just hide from you. You often will not see me on my bad days. I hide away because it is embarrassing and frustrating to try to function in a fast-paced world with a slow-processing brain. Brain injury is already a lonely world, made lonelier by hiding away, because it is all just too much to tolerate. If an award was given for the best actress pretending to feel okay, I like to think I'd be a shoo-in.

Before I go any further, let me preface this by saying that my pain is very high right now, which means my patience is low. I have not responded to any pain medications since August. When I say, "responded to," that does not mean the pain was gone because it is never gone, but it was tolerable. I can function with it and can fake my smile easier. Living with high levels of pain, day-after-day, week-after-week, month-after-month, is draining. This is something that I would never wish on anybody.

> ## Like many others, I hide what I am going through a lot.

For those who struggle to understand what they cannot see; for those that read my words but they still don't sink in, and for those that have romanticized the idea of a brain injury and think it's a relaxing vacation, I'd like to set the record straight.

It is impossible to put it all into words. It would take me months to write down every little thing that I go through. Let's face it, no one would read that. I do, however, need to try to draw some awareness to this life, a life that I did not ask for, a life that few people would have wished for themselves.

It has been thirty-nine months since the accident. Thirty-nine long, lonely, frustrating, and painful months. In those months, I have consumed more medications than I have in the thirty-five years prior. I have been more frustrated, tired, emotional, stressed, angry, sad, and in more pain than I ever thought possible. In spite of this, I try not to forget that it could be so much worse.

You cannot shut off a brain injury. It is always with you. Daily I live with sensitivity to light and noise, pain and over-stimulation – both visually and auditory. You do not know tired until you know brain injury tired. Keep in mind that this is coming from a teacher! I used to think "end-of-school-year-teacher tired" was hard enough. You need tough skin because you might be the butt of many jokes. Some days I can laugh at myself with you, but in reality, it feels like I have just been punched. You need to battle with family and friends that say to you, "I can't possibly understand what you're going through." Although that statement is completely accurate, there is nothing that says you cannot try to understand. In reality, you can ask questions or do some research. I am always happy to answer questions, just don't minimize what I say or respond with, "Oh yeah, I get headaches too."

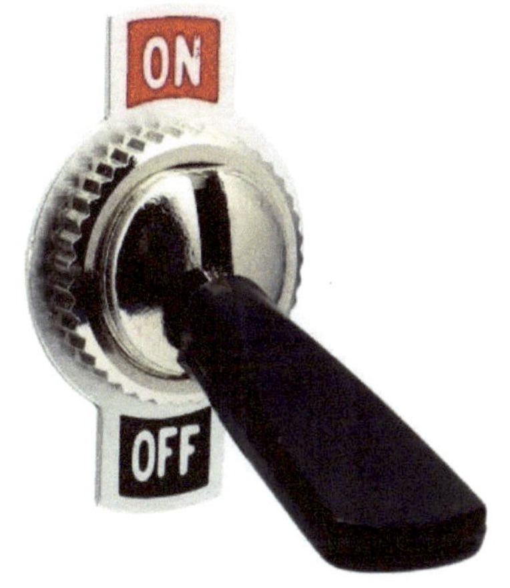

You cannot shut off a brain injury. It is always with you.

I had a doctor once ask me how much sleep I get at night. Letting him know I averaged twelve hours a night, he replied, "Must be nice. I wish I could sleep that much." My reply blindsided him. "Get hit by a car and you can!"

Well-intentioned friends say things like, "I forget things too," or "I've had a headache all morning and I want to die." It is just not the same for those of us living with a brain injury. I've actually had people mock me when my words fail like, "t-t-t-today." I've had people make jokes at my expense when I say the wrong word like, "I take magazine at night." In my head, I said "I take melatonin at night." I've received funny looks when I draw a blank mid-conversation wondering what we were talking about. I've wanted to walk away from my shopping cart in the store because I literally CANNOT handle one more noise or one more visually stimulating thing, causing my brain to virtually shut down. Yet, even if you walk away from that cart, the noise, the visual stimulation still remains. Cars passing by, buildings in the distance, traffic lights… I often feel like the Grinch. "There's one thing I can't stand...all the noise, noise, noise, noise!"

Just today, my day started at 3:00 AM. My head hurt so much that I could not get comfortable. Finally, around 7:00 AM, I was able to fall back to sleep. This disruption in my sleep can have harsh consequences. I slept off and on until the afternoon, before I needed to rise and get ready to make the trek in the freezing rain, down to my neurologist's office. Just getting ready was exhausting enough, but it's not like I could go back to sleep. I needed to travel to Dartmouth. Once at the doctors, she reviews my "daily headache chart" and just shakes her head. Nothing is working. What do we do next? We try yet another medication and like so many before, this medication comes with a warning I must heed: "this medication will make you sick! So, ease into it." All these pills, these shots/injections just to try to make it so I can function with never-ending pain.

Why in the world would anyone say to me "I wish I was you!"? Because they don't understand that life with a brain injury is more complicated than anyone will ever know. It is my hope that some might now better understand that which they cannot see.

Meet Jen Dodge

Jen is a resident of northern New Hampshire. On August 19, 2014, she was hit by an SUV while riding her bicycle on a group ride. Since the accident she has written several articles titled "Confessions of a Concussed Cyclist" to help inform others and as a form of therapy for herself. She is a certified Special Education teacher, and an avid cyclist. Jen uses her own story to encourage people to become informed about the invisible disability of a brain injury and to be kind to cyclists and Share the Road!

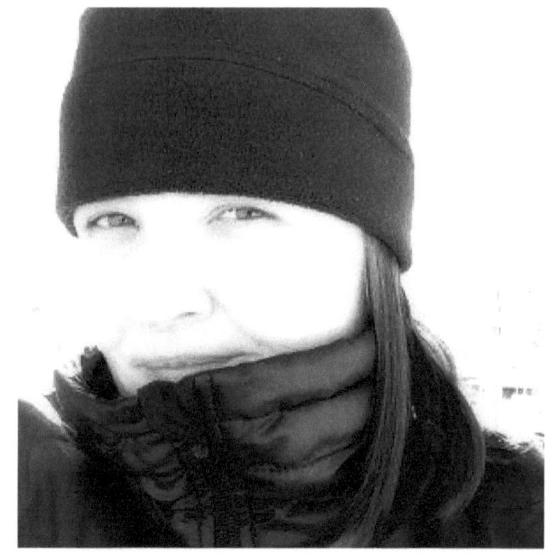

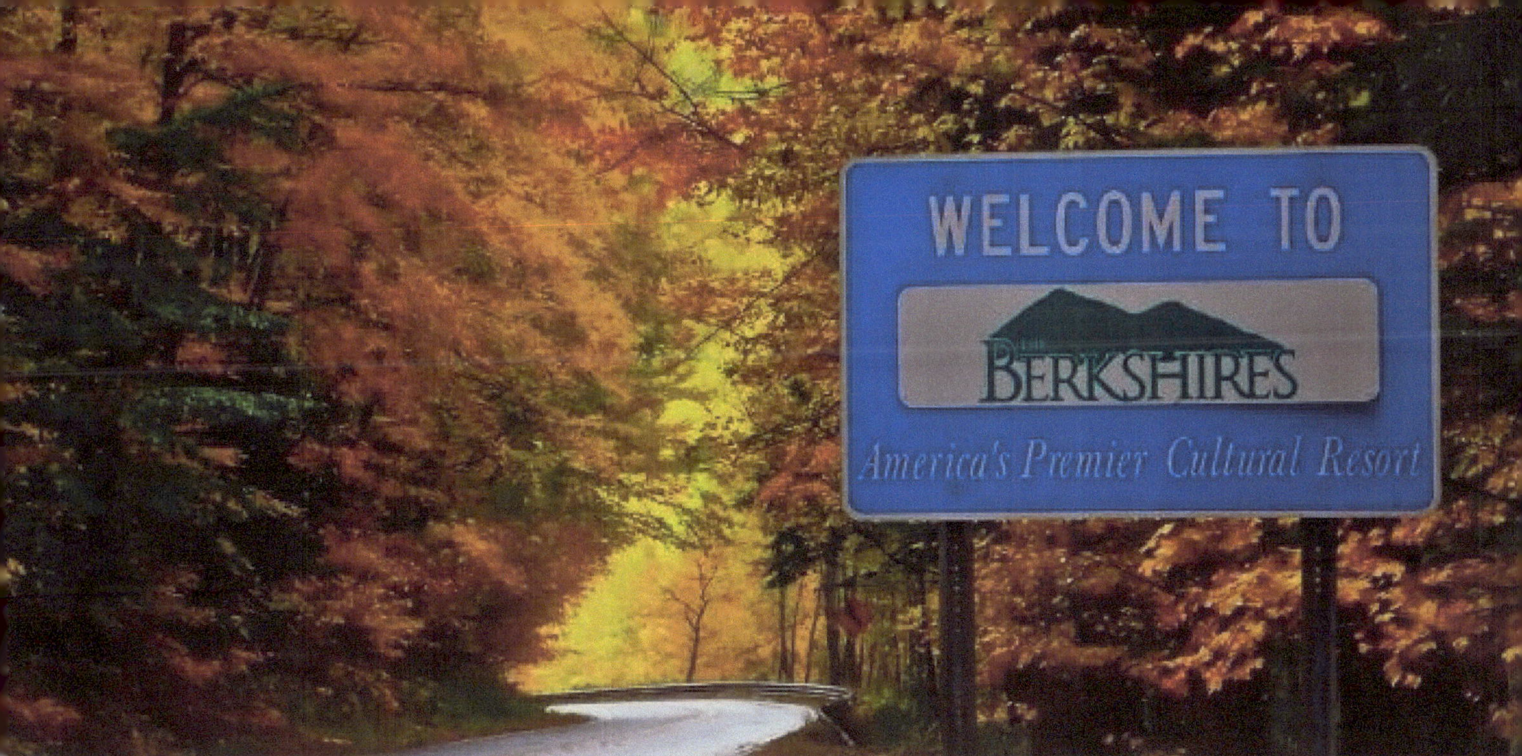

The Glass Box

By Stacia Bissell

I suppose every brain injury survivor views his or her own struggle and story a little differently than the next. After I suffered my traumatic brain injury in 2011, my pre-injury and post-injury lives became clearly delineated and I began regarding my body as host to two distinct versions of me that still act like strangers today.

Version Two is sitting down penning this article after another migrainous day spent primarily alone, while soothing my aching head into submission using many clever techniques that are neither scientific nor consistent from one achy episode to the next. Version One is someone I now perceive to be sitting down while looking straight at me through my own familiar light grayish-blue eyes from within a crystal-clear, tightly sealed shatterproof glass box. One might question whether I am simply mistaking the insular glass box for a mirror, but the lack of synchronicity between the abilities and behaviors of these two women tell me otherwise.

I remember my pre-injury self as being confident, poised, professional, well-dressed, in control, with a long to-do list and the capability of accomplishing everything on it - and then some. She was on a mission to prove herself in many areas of her life and she was a bit of workaholic. She could look out and pretty clearly see where she was heading personally and professionally. Under the surface of the more serious woman in the glass box was a fun, spirited girl who enjoyed family time, social time and alone time. She was a good mom, attentive wife, daughter and friend, and someone who cared deeply about the people she worked with and the 100 plus students who came through her classroom doors every day in a busy middle school. Although my pre-injury self goes wherever I go, she is now parked quietly inside a transparent cube with the access road to her closed.

On September 2, 2011, I fell from my bicycle and suffered a broken arm, some road rash and a life-altering brain injury, while riding with a friend along a scenic bike trail in the Berkshires in western Massachusetts. The moment of contact between my helmet and the pavement (yes, I was wearing a helmet) was the instant that Version One was boxed up in a shiny glass container and the seams tightly secured, and this new version of me, Version Two, began breathing and existing.

In the early darkness of my brain injury, a blurry, confused, emotional, tired STRANGER tried accessing the old me in the glass box. I could see Version One; I could hear her, remember her, and recall the things she could accomplish in a day's time with a busy family and a full-time job. But there she sat dormant. I'd set out to act like her, perform tasks like her and talk like her, but what I ended up actually doing and saying was foreign. Although I used to be a fabulous cook, I no longer knew how to make even a grilled cheese sandwich or pancakes. I found that I now stuttered and misplaced or misused words, and that I sometimes said things that sounded more like they came from a truck driver's mouth than mine. Sometimes I'd make a to-do list in the morning and find that I could only manage taking a shower that day before fatigue, head pain and confusion would set it off and I'd have to rest and hope for a more productive day the next day.

I acquired a neurologist after my fall, among other specialists, and she told me that I couldn't work, couldn't drive, and had to take a lineup of medications for sleep issues, chronic headaches and depression; three things that I didn't have an issue with up to that particular day in September. My world and social life began being measured by doctors' appointments and the people I would talk to when I got there. Every day I would persistently pound on the box thinking that if I banged hard enough, then that familiar-looking person inside would emerge, and life would go back to normal instead of me leading this unfamiliar life.

> **My world and social life began being measured by doctors' appointments and the people I would talk to when I got there.**

About four months after my accident, my speech language pathologist, Katya Bowen, told me that I might recover more if I would stop fighting my injury, start accepting it and begin working hard at managing it. That was the day that I sat up and started paying closer attention to the strategies that she was teaching me in order to do simple, every day things again, like find a number in a phone book, clean my house, plan and sequence my day, find items in a grocery store, or go out successfully in social settings.

It was at this point that I also made the decision to become as knowledgeable as I could about brain injury, and to understand the nuances of my own specific set of post-concussion particulars. I began reading, researching and asking a lot of questions. One year later, I was finally able to return to work full time. After working for only twenty-four months in that setting, a doctor pulled me due to the adverse and accumulated effect that working in that setting was having on my recovery.

The period of time after this juncture was difficult for me because a large chunk of my identity was lost, on top of many other significant losses I was already faced with. However, it was also the point that I began feeling physically stronger, attended my first brain injury support group, and kicked off a journey to educate others about brain injury and be a voice when other survivors cannot. I have had opportunities to speak at conferences, corporate staff meetings, on television, and for civic and non-profit organizations.

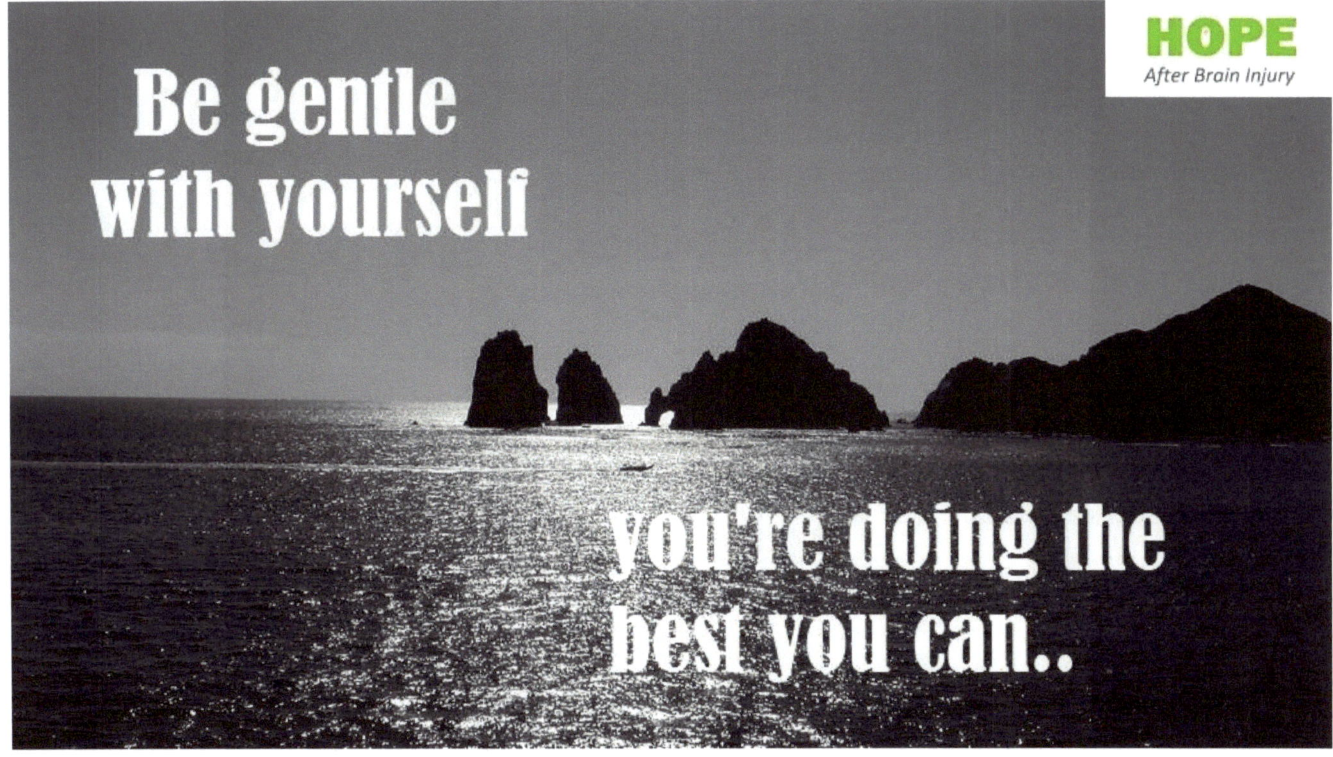

Sometimes I am the sole speaker sharing my story, while at other times, my former SLP, Katya, joins me on stage for added value and comic relief. I am a founding member of the Berkshire Brain Injury Collaborative, which provides professional development to educators with return-to-learn strategies to help students who have suffered from a concussion, and I co-founded and continue to co-facilitate a monthly brain injury support group in Northampton, Massachusetts.

I thought I would have to get 100% better before I could have a future where good things could come my way. But, I found instead that with this sort of disability, you adapt to a new life while your dreams and goals simultaneously begin adapting to you. Eventually, I learned to stop searching so hard for missing pieces and aimed instead to find the misplaced peace that came with other losses.

While I lost many relationships since 2011, including the easy conformity I had with the woman in the glass box, my husband of 25 years, some friends, and a career I loved, I thankfully learned how to make and sustain meaningful new relationships. I've now learned how to slow down and be grateful, how to prioritize things more clearly, how to grow some of my own food, and take care of a house and yard without too much help. Camping, hiking, kayaking and biking are still things I enjoy, and I've learned to say yes to new things like public speaking, zip lining and flying in a 4-seater plane. I've *finally* learned to say no. And I've also learned to say "No way!" to an expiration date on my recovery. Who knows, maybe one of these days a small crack will appear in the glass box.

Meet Stacia Bissell

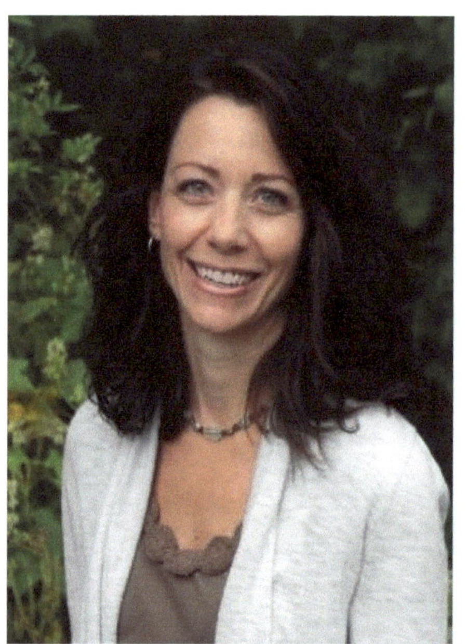

Stacia Bissell is a native of Berkshire County in Western Massachusetts. She studied mathematics at Wells College in Aurora, New York and earned a Master's in Education degree from Cambridge College. Passionate about education, Stacia spent much of her career as a middle school math teacher and high school business teacher until taking on roles in administration and academic coaching. In 2011 her career as a public school educator came to an end.

With encouragement from the Brain Injury Association of Massachusetts, friends and family, Stacia began doing speaking engagements to various audiences on the topic of brain injury. In addition to being a keynote speaker for a number of organizations, she is a co-facilitator of the Northampton Brain Injury Support Group and a founding member of the Berkshire Brain Injury Collaborative.

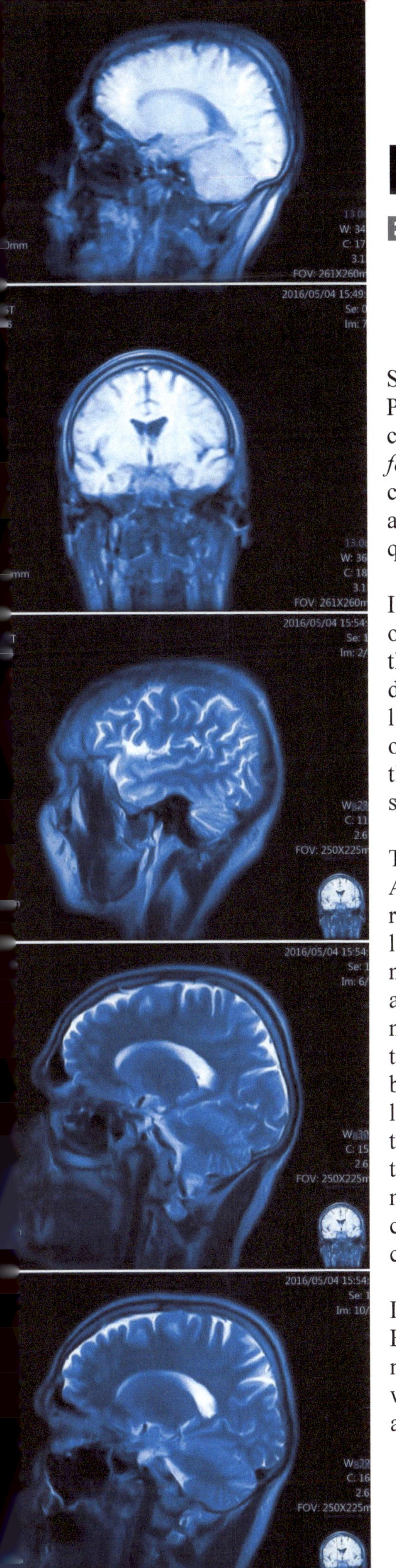

Living with an AVM
By Paul McMonagle

Seventeen years ago, I was diagnosed with a genetic brain disorder. Prior to my diagnosis, I had never heard of an AVM. Is this brain condition an *"irregular, anomalous, abnormal, or faulty formation or structure"* as defined by the medical community? I have asked that question to myself, my family, and my doctors. Most importantly, I asked my God that question.

If this condition was nothing I could have planned, affected, or caused, then why did it happen to me? And if you go down that line of thinking, you will end up in a very dark and depressing place. So, over the last seventeen years that I've lived with this condition, it rather has been a great opportunity to see the grace, the care, the hope, and the love that both has been given to me and is given among those who suffer similar conditions.

The condition of an AVM is one largely shrouded in mystery. AVM's form based on some incorrect gene instructions regarding the construction of faulty blood vessels. It is largely fatal when occurring inside the skull. What should it mean if you have this disorder? Well, rather than lose hope and find despair, I *hope* that you will see it as a gift. This may sound strange, but hear me out. If you are alive to read this, then you have survived up until now, with this disorder besetting you. Moreover, you have lots of questions that are largely unanswered. The medical community is diligently trying to find cures and treatments for this condition. From traditional open cranium craniotomy (been there), to the more futuristic gamma knife procedure (been there too, very cool setup), embolization and others, treatments are changing.

I grew up in southeast Alabama, graduated from New Brockton High, and went off to Auburn. But in pursuit of a new life following my brain bleed, I had to relearn how to walk, talk, read, and write. It was tremendously challenging and at times heartbreaking.

Nevertheless, post-injury, I was able to meet the woman of my dreams, father two of the most beautiful children in the world, finish my bachelors, masters, and education specialist degrees, and meet so many friends and colleagues as we traveled on.

The message of encouragement I hope to share with this world is simply this: you are here for a specific purpose. You did not arrive by chance, you weren't even born by accident. You have a purpose on this earth. If I had not experienced an initial brain bleed in the apartment of my girlfriend at the time at Auburn, I would not have enrolled in DBU where I met my wife Leslie.

If we had not pursued trying to have a child in spite of the doctors advising that it would likely never happen, we would not have had our first daughter. If I had not lost my job in Dothan, I would never have been asked to serve as pastor of a church for five years where we were blessed by the birth of another daughter.

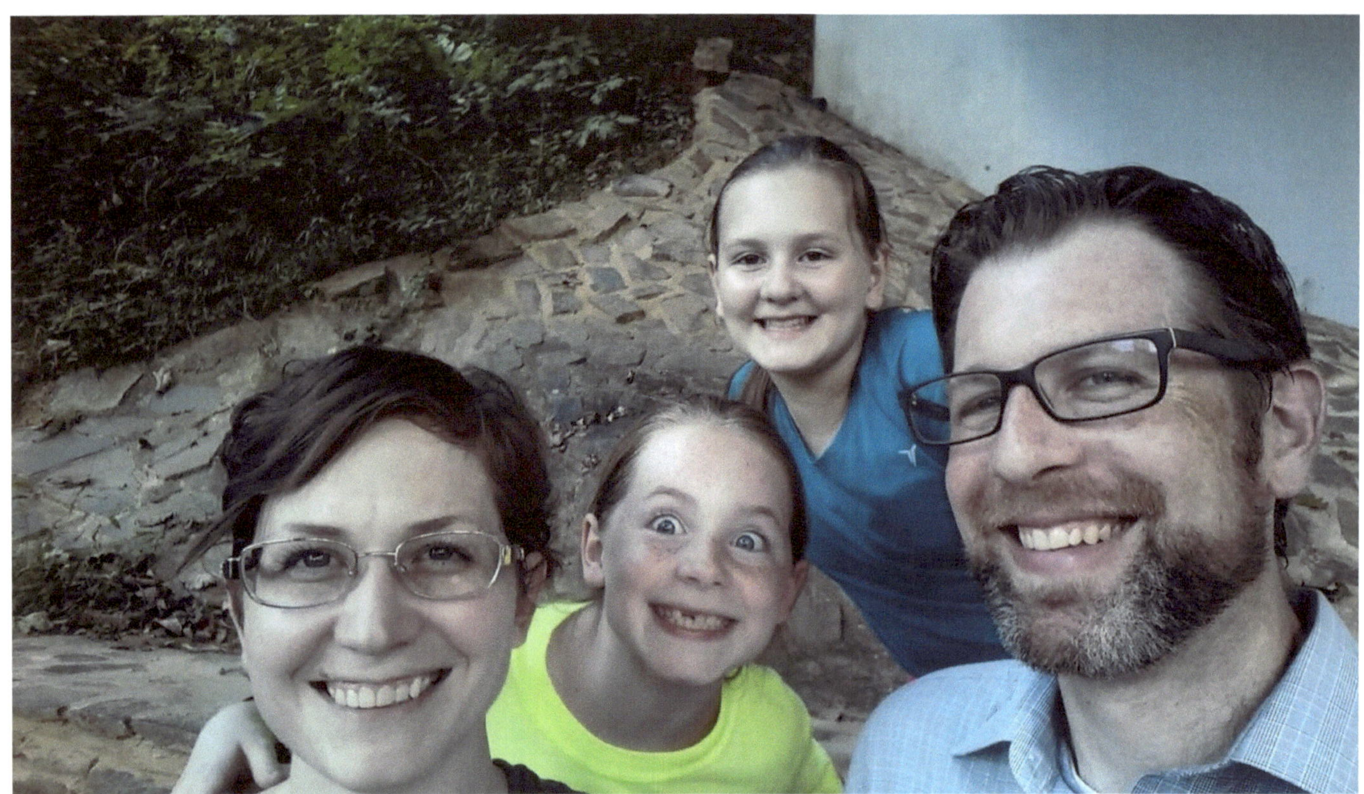

If I had not pursued further education, our family would never have known the friends and family we have now. Life truly is a process not a destination. The only destination our bodies are all sure to end up is the grave. So, in the interim between life and death, my challenge is to live to the best of my abilities. Sure, those abilities change as time goes on, but until those abilities are all used up, I will shine a light.

There are three things I want to do as a brain injured person. First, I want to impart hope to the hurting. Do not let the fact that you suffer with this condition be the end of your life. Rather, see it as an adventure. You will have to ask for help, but surround yourself with groups of persons who have similar struggles to see that you're not alone. This isn't a plug for a specific church, but as a former pastor I can say, nowhere else will I find in the community such a collection of persons from all walks of life dealing with all sorts of issues that I can both learn from and speak hope into their lives.

Second, our family has a fun time searching for things anyway. Why not make a game of it? Think of it as a manual Amazon Alexa or Google Home. Our children are awesome at asking questions, why not use that as an opportunity to ask them questions in turn. If they are like mine, they'll respond. Often when it is time to do house chores or laundry, I will turn it into a sort of game or contest. This takes the drudgery out of the mundane and instead transforms it into an adventure. Revisiting the parts of life that seemed to blow by so quickly can be a useful tool at highlighting the mistakes that might have otherwise been missed.

Third, and perhaps the most important, is to recognize you are still here. I cannot stress that enough. If you are still here, regardless of how you feel, you are still here. That means something! Your survival in this tragedy means that you were not taken. That fact in and of itself is worth celebrating, but I would guess that there are other persons in your life right now who are pleased that you're alive as well. Do not give up hope! Rest in knowing there are others like yourself and the future only gets brighter!

Meet Paul McMonagle

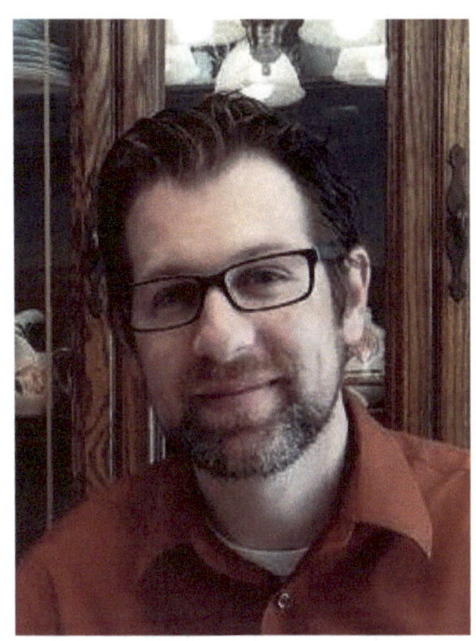

Paul McMonagle and his wife Leslie currently live in Lynchburg, Virginia. A proud father, among his many blessings, he considers his life to be blessed by his girls, his wife, and his church family. Paul is also a former pastor at the Rocky Head Baptist Church in Ariton, Alabama.

In addition to his passion for life and serving others, Paul is a regular writer and blogger. You can read Paul's blog at: www.malformationblog.wordpress.com

All we have to decide is what to do with the time that is given us.

~J.R.R. Tolkien

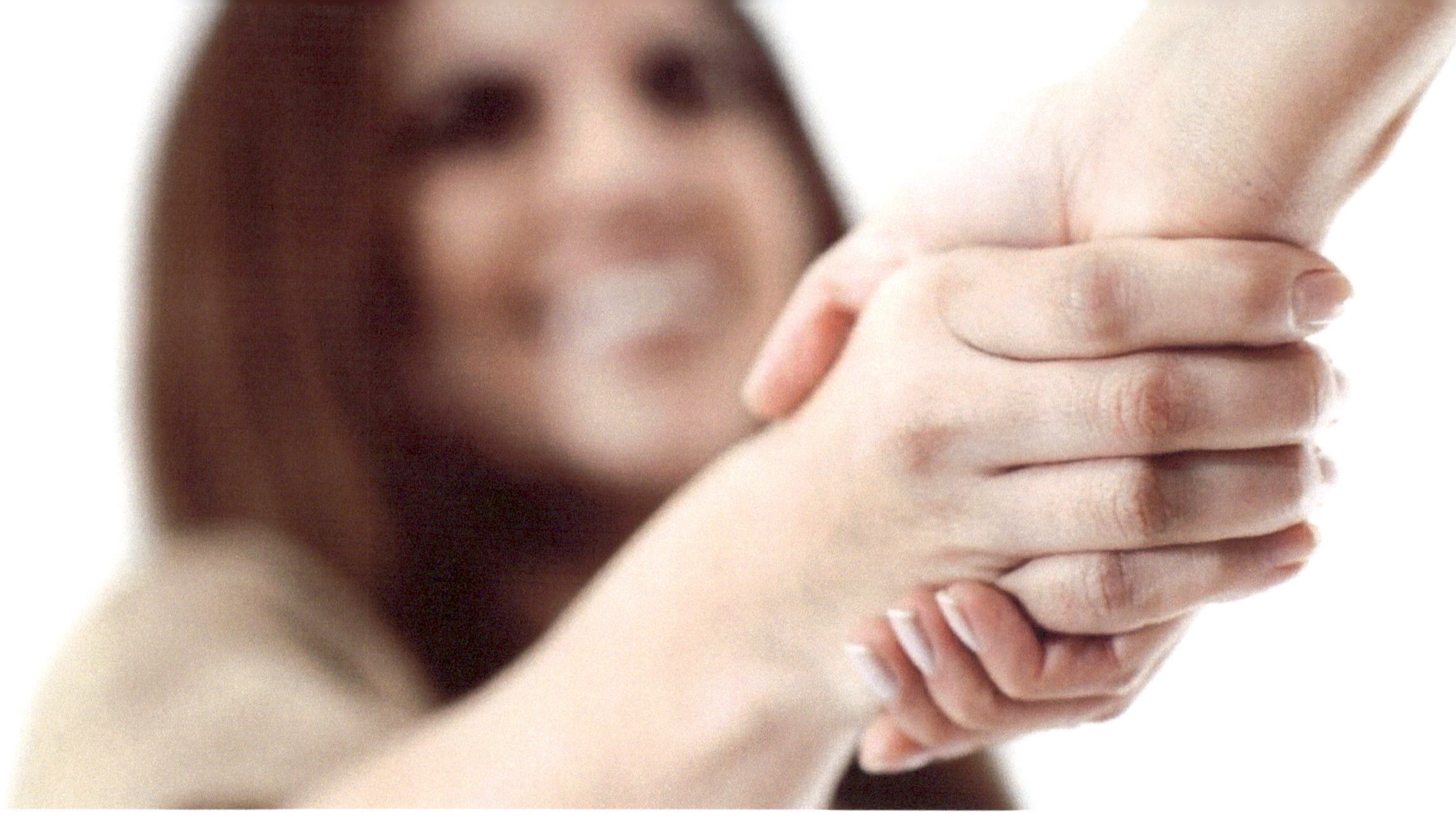

Finding a Job After Brain Injury

By Donna O'Donnell Figurski

Everything is running smoothly in your life. You may have a job you like or love, or maybe you hate it but, still, you have a job. A job provides a sense of accomplishment and a feeling of responsibility and independence.

Many folks take pride in their jobs or careers. In fact, "What do you do?" is one of the first questions we all ask folks we meet for the first time. For some, like me, it's curiosity. I love to find folks who have the same interests as I do. I score when I find another elementary-school teacher or someone who works in the theater, or another jewelry-crafter. I can talk for hours on those topics. So, sometimes people just want to know because they are curious.

> **"What do you do?" is one of the first questions we all ask folks we meet for the first time.**

But other times, folks ask as a means to measure up with others. They want to see where their job falls on the job-ladder-of-success.

Either way, it seems that having a job is very important to folks. It not only provides the monies to support oneself and one's family but, in this time when jobs are hard to get, it definitely provides a sense of achievement.

When a person has a brain injury, that person's brain may not work well enough to return to his or her former job. In fact, it may be difficult for survivors to retain any job.

A survivor of brain injury may suffer a number of disabilities that could interfere with job performance. Extreme fatigue, memory loss, or emotional or behavioral issues could easily cause disruption and interfere in a normal work-day. Many survivors have sustained physical injury with their brain injury. Disabilities, like compromised sight, lack-of-balance, ataxic hands, or any number of other physical afflictions, may impede a survivor from adequately performing a job.

Having no job and not being a productive part of society can pose a myriad of problems for survivors, often lowering their self-esteem. These can add to the complications that life has already wreaked on them and, again, that question - "What do you do?" - looms.

Survivors with no job may sense a lack of purpose in their lives, which can easily cause them to feel embarrassed or worthless or even to become depressed. With no job, paying the bills that are due each month becomes an all-encompassing worry. For many, it may be as daunting as climbing the 16,000-foot-high Mount Kilimanjaro. Needless to say, it is problematic when there is little money to cover the basic needs of food, clothing, and shelter. Survivors often feel that they've become a burden to their family members, especially those survivors who once were entirely independent and now must return home for care.

A survivor-friend of mine once said, "I am still me but, at the same time, I am not." That's a very insightful statement. She realized that, though she is still the same person in her mind, she has limitations. When a survivor comes to grips with what he or she is able to adequately do or to accomplish, that survivor is headed in the right direction. When survivors pine over their lost life and strive to regain that pre-injury life, which understandably so many do, it seems to take them longer to grasp their new selves and move on with their new capabilities.

> **When a survivor comes to grips with what he or she is able to adequately do or to accomplish, that survivor is headed in the right direction**

That's not to say to give up or surrender to the brain injury, but rather to focus on what is now attainable and forge ahead.

So, what can a survivor do to overcome this challenge? How can he or she find a productive job and prosper in it?

There is no advice that will be a one-size-fits-all, just as there are no two brain injury survivors with the same brain injury. So, the survivor must assess his or her own capabilities - perhaps with the help of family and/or friends. Also, doctors or therapists who know the strengths and weaknesses of the survivor may be welcome assets. As a survivor, make a list of the things you like to do. If you are personable and like to help people, you might want to get a job working in a home-improvement store or a small boutique. If you are techy, perhaps an office-supply store that sells computers and other electronics would interest you. If you are the quiet type, maybe you could work in a small office. If you have an aversion to loud noises and/or bright lights, you may want to avoid jobs in sports bars and restaurants. Only you can decide what would work best for you.

What can a survivor of brain injury do if he or she is not able to find and adequately perform a job? That happens all too often. If the injury is so debilitating that it prevents the survivor from holding any kind of responsible job, he or she may possibly want to pursue a volunteer position with less restrictions on hours and commitment. Though no money will exchange hands, the payment is bountiful with smiles, accomplishments, feelings of pride, and social interactions.

Volunteering in a nursing home, an animal-rescue site, or a food-pantry can provide immense satisfaction. Local libraries or YMCA's often need volunteers. There are many places. Perform a Google search for volunteer sites in your area and see what opportunities are available. You will not only be helping others, you will be helping yourself.

If you simply cannot obtain a paying job, you may want to consider disability from Social Security. Getting approved is not always easy, and you may have to apply more than once, but don't be discouraged.

Life after brain injury is not easy. Finding a job or some kind of work/volunteer placement will no doubt be challenging, but with patience and persistence and maybe a little creative thinking, you can find some enriching opportunities to enhance your life. I hope so!

Meet Donna O'Donnell Figurski

Donna O'Donnell Figurski, is a wife, mother, granny, teacher, playwright, actor, director, picture-book reviewer, radio host, speaker, photographer, and writer. As a brain-injury advocate, Donna has published articles in many brain-injury-related magazines on the web; has written chapters for two books, and writes a brain injury blog. Donna resides in the desert with her husband and best friend, David, who had a traumatic brain injury in 2005.

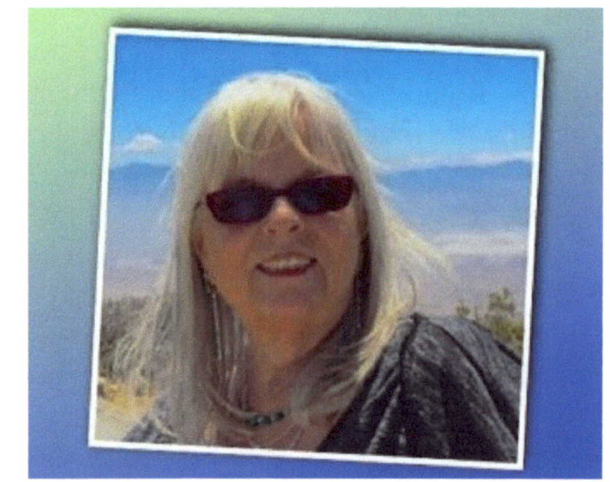

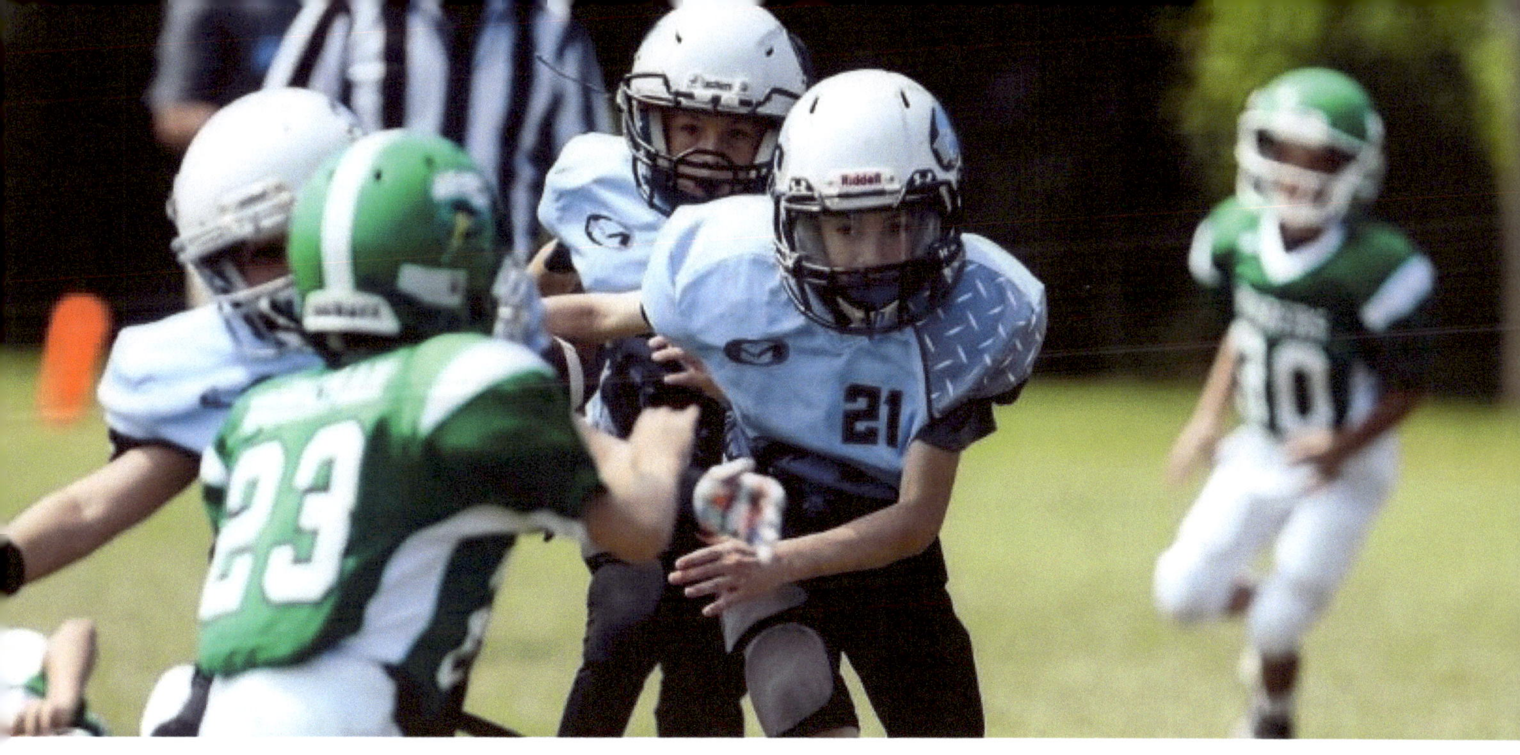

The Human League
By Ted Stachulski

In the fall of 1986, after my suicide attempt, I was sent back to high school without an Individual Education Plan (IEP) or any speech or occupational therapy for the multitude of concussions I had suffered from playing contact sports. I found out a family member and a friend met with the Superintendent of Schools to see if he would allow me to be a senior that school year and graduate with my class. Their plea was denied and I had to repeat my junior year.

I found myself back on the high school football team. It was more of a matter of habit than actually wanting to be there. The new head coach looked at me and made me a running back. I had played the position many years prior in Pop Warner football, but I had spent most of my time since then as an offensive guard, defensive tackle, and a special team's player.

I had other issues to deal with such as my teammates who were angry with me for things I had done on and off the field. The previous year I had quit the team after the last regular season game heading into the playoffs because of a Second Impact Syndrome and then I engaged in risky behavior that put others in danger.

It was not hard to tell they wanted revenge and I had a target on my back. On the way to the practice field they would yell out, "It's a great day to be alive!" mocking my suicide attempt. During practice, I was the running back who ran plays against the starting defense. It was only a matter of time before the second string offensive line collapsed and I was dead meat in the backfield. I was gang tackled and blew out my right knee. Revenge was had.

I continued to go to practices and games, but I stayed on the sidelines because I was on crutches. I began to notice the benefits of not hitting and banging my head every day playing football. I had more attention, focus, and less mental fatigue, I did not have the usual difficulty with schoolwork or a slump in my grades and I was looking for ways to build relationships instead of letting impulsivity, depression, anxiety and aggression ruin relationships.

The Centers for Disease Control (CDC) defines a traumatic brain injury (TBI) as a disruption in the normal function of the brain that can be caused by a bump, blow, or jolt to the head, or penetrating head injury. According to the CDC, an estimated 2.8 million people sustain a traumatic brain injury annually. 52,000 die, 282,000 are hospitalized and 2.5 million are treated and released from an emergency department.

A TBI can cause epilepsy and increase the risk for conditions such as Alzheimer's disease, Parkinson's disease, and other brain disorders.

Approximately 75% of TBIs that occur each year are concussions or other forms of mild TBI.

Repeated mild TBIs occurring over an extended period can result in cumulative neurological and cognitive deficits. Repeated mild TBIs occurring within a short period (i.e., hours, days, or weeks) can be catastrophic or fatal.

According to the Boston University CTE Center, Chronic Traumatic Encephalopathy (CTE) is a progressive degenerative disease of the brain found in athletes (and others) with a history of repetitive brain trauma, including symptomatic concussions as well as asymptomatic subconcussive hits to the head.

I was relieved the superintendent denied the request to be a senior because what I needed most was time. I needed time to rest my brain after school and to retake and pass the classes I had failed the year before. I needed time to deal with the demons of Post-Concussion Syndrome and to focus on building relationships while leaving the macho attitude behind. I needed time to address my alcohol and pain pill addictions, and I needed time to reconnect with my community and share what I had been through.

But how was I going to accomplish all of this?

Fortunately for me, a guidance counselor and a teacher were trying to get a new school program off the ground called Peer Outreach. Knowing I was in deep trouble emotionally and physically, they took me and other challenged at-risk high school students under their wings in order to train us to share our stories with younger students in the community. The Peer Outreach Program allowed me to meet students from other New Hampshire high schools who were survivors of the circumstances that affected their lives. We were given an opportunity to open up to one another about our terrible experiences and great friendships were formed.

During a Peer Outreach training retreat, I met a girl from another town. Her name was Melissa. We were polar opposites in every way but attracted to each other just the same. We spent time together whenever we could and our friendship grew. She was there for me at the right time with the right knowledge and friendship to help me move on from football and concussions.

One Saturday morning I was at her house. She knew I had a football game and asked me, "Why are you here and not at the game?"

It was because being with her was like being in a Human League vs. being in a Sports League. It was a very different way of life than I was used to and I was fascinated by the way she lived and what her priorities were. There were not any contact sports, games, practices, repetitive collisions or concussions and she showed me there was actually a world where I didn't have to repeatedly bash my brain against my skull to get ahead. That I could be still in both body and mind, eat well, exercise safely in moderation and enjoy the here and now.

I was used to going to ball fields and parks to kick and throw balls, run and think about my future. Instead, she held my hand while we sat still, meditated and lived in the present moment.

I was poor and used to shopping at local discount stores. She took me to the outlet stores in Freeport, Maine. I was used to surviving off school lunches for nutrition so she took me to fancy restaurants. I used to skip school with my friends to ride the Boston subway system and end up in places like the combat zone. She drove me to Boston in her car on the weekend and took me to places like the Museum of Fine Art. I always wore athletic apparel and in the winter I wore heavy sweatshirts and sweatpants. She bought me a nice wool coat to keep warm. I had trophies, medals, and ribbons hanging on my bedroom walls. She had framed Ansel Adams pictures hanging from her walls. While I talked about going into the military after high school, she talked about SAT's and going to college after high school.

> **I was poor and used to shopping at local discount stores. She took me to the outlet stores in Freeport, Maine. I was used to surviving off school lunches for nutrition so she took me to fancy restaurants.**

My priorities changed and my focus was now on academics, relationship building, and fitness. To make up the credits I needed to graduate high school, I had a class every period and took classes at night. It was hard at first, but as time went on I found a groove and stuck with it. When the time was right, I began running several miles per day and lifting weights again. My Uncle David was a Marine Corps recruiter and I got to PT and drill with his Poolies.

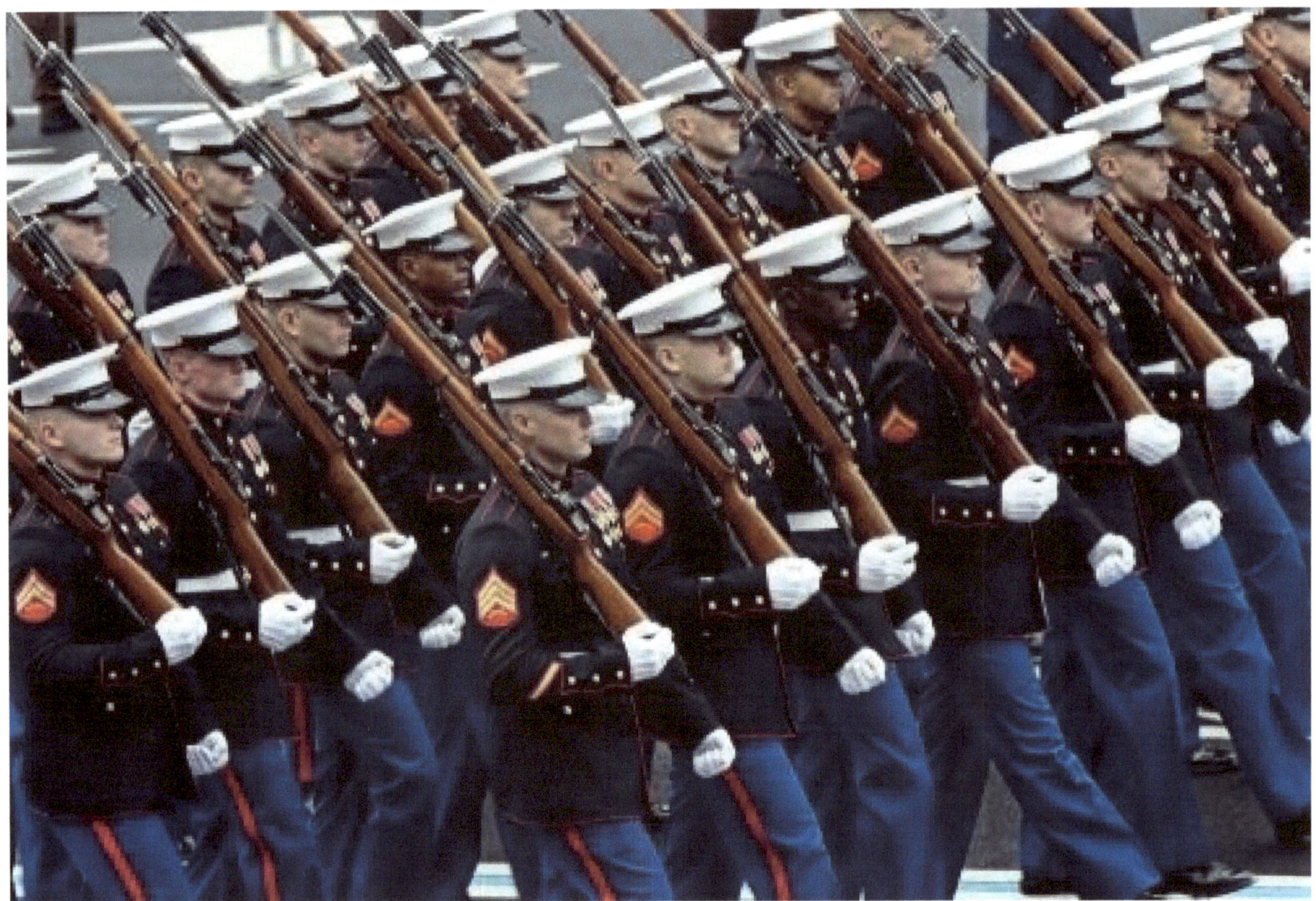

Eventually, the time came where I had to bid farewell to Melissa. I had enough credits to graduate high school and I joined the United States Marine Corps. When my name was called to receive my high school diploma at graduation, I was over a thousand miles away attending Marine Corps boot camp in Parris Island, South Carolina. Ever since I was a little boy I wanted to follow in the footsteps of many of my relatives who served in the military.

Not once did I ever dream of playing college, minor league or professional sports. Never in my wildest dreams would I have ever thought that contact sports could have delayed or prevented me from going into the military.

A decade's worth of repeated blows and multiple sports concussions were not necessary to become a man or a Marine and the long-term effects of them hurt me every step of the way in my military career. It occurred to me that military service members with prior sports concussions could possibly have a negative effect on the battlefield if they sustained another traumatic brain injury in combat.

I was not the first or the last recruit to join the military having had multiple sports concussions. In an interview on July 25, 2014, Retired Army General Peter Chiarelli explained, "But that was one of the huge issues that we saw in the Army was that most of our folks came into the Army having already suffered concussions from playing football, lacrosse, soccer and other kinds of contact sports."

I lost contact with Melissa for almost thirty years and recently reconnected with her on Facebook. I was glad to find out she graduated college and has been working as a Clinical Social Worker. As for me, according to my VA Neurologist, my "presentation and history is entirely consistent with severe post-concussion syndrome (or worse) with permanent neurobehavioral sequelae."

For over a decade I've been sharing my traumatic brain injury experience with Veterans, athletes and their family members and helping them improve the quality of their lives as Melissa helped improve mine so many years ago. Thank you, Melissa!

Meet Ted Stachulski

Ted Stachulski is a former multi-sport athlete, Marine Corps Veteran, Traumatic Brain Injury Survivor, creator of the Veterans Traumatic Brain Injury Survivor Guide. Ted is also a Veterans Outreach Specialist and an advocate for brain injury survivors, their family members and caregivers. You can learn more about Ted at www.TBITed.com

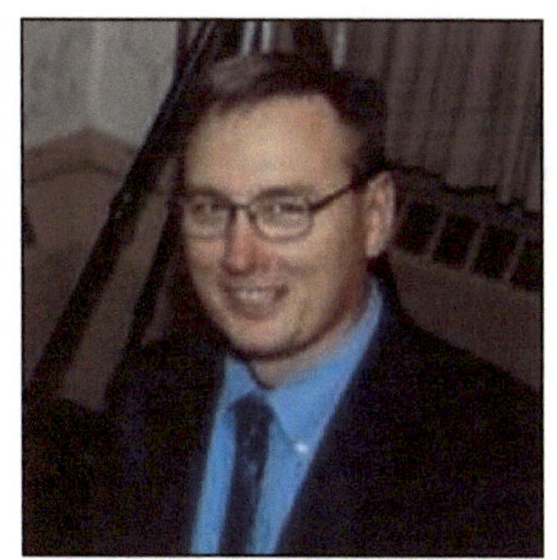

INTRODUCING THE NEW
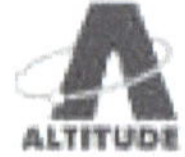 dish FLEX PACK

Create Your Own TV Package

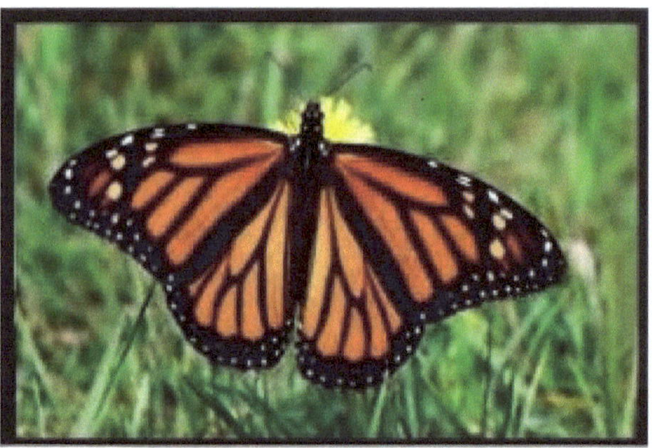

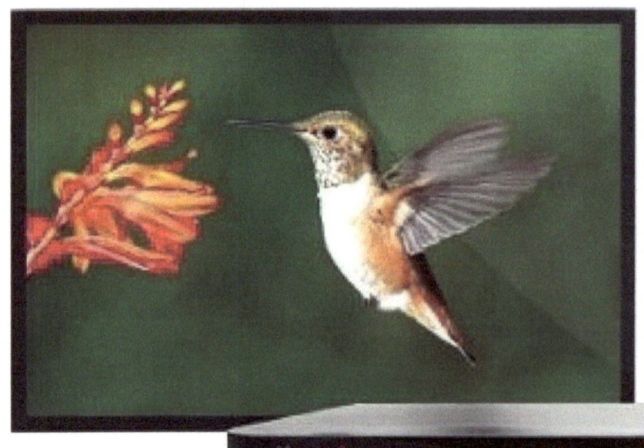

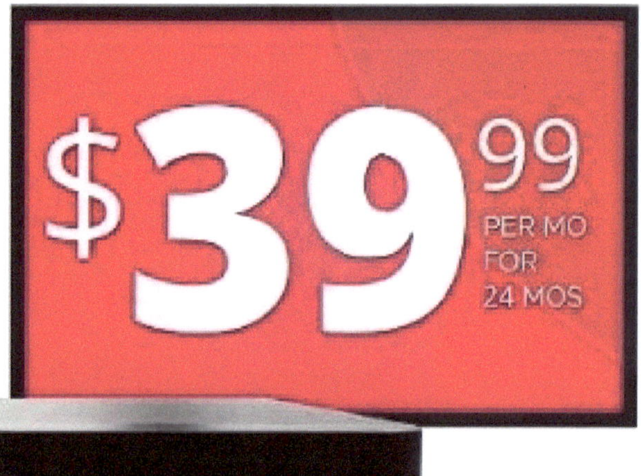

Free Streaming   **Free Installation**   **Add Internet**

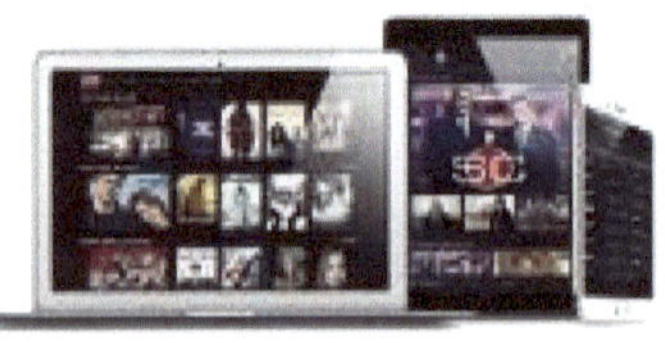

+

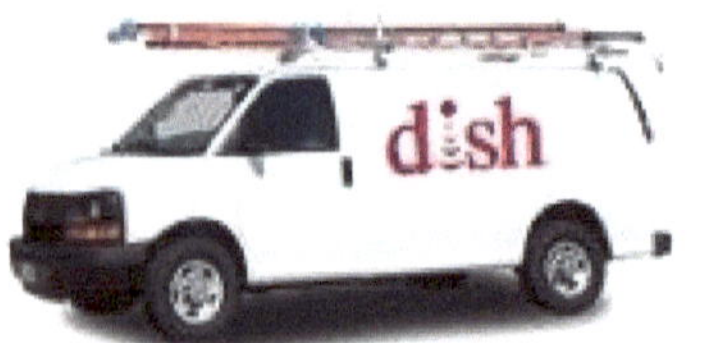

+

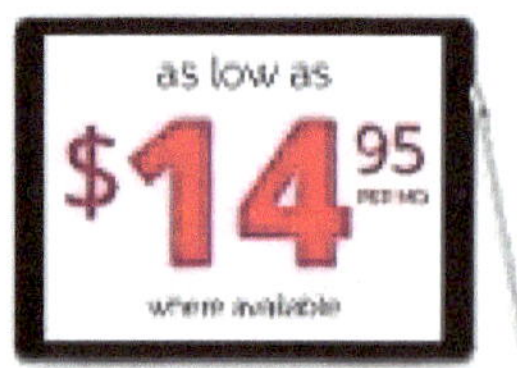

Call 1-800-391-1328

News & Views

The end of one year marks the beginning of another. While I am not a fan of New Year's Resolutions, I do like to set goals. Very often, resolutions involve trying to get away from something unhealthy. "This year, I'll eat less junk food," or "Starting in 2018, I'll spend less time on the couch." Goals, however, are something to strive toward. That being said, in 2018, I have set a rather interesting goal, the goal of doing less.

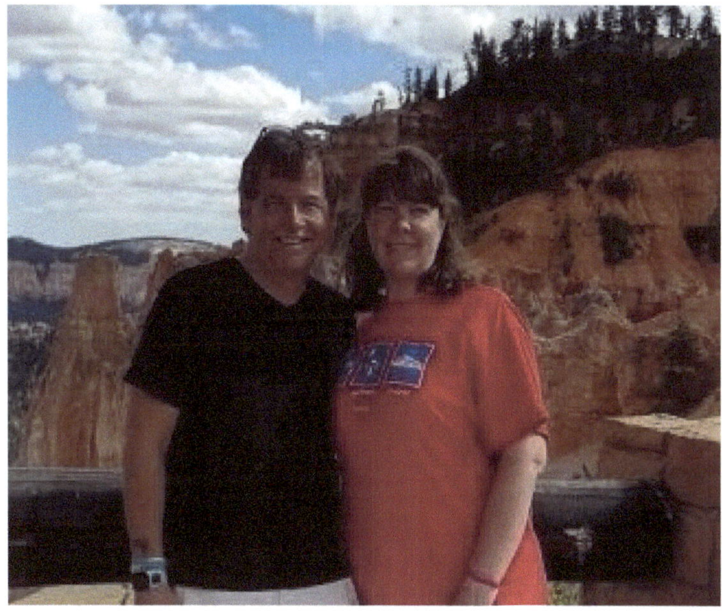

Let me explain. A couple of years ago, an organizational leader shared that his organization as *"a mile wide and an inch deep."* Though many projects were on the table, it was hard to delve deep into any one of them. I am an overachiever by nature. Early on in my recovery, I wanted to set the world on fire, advocating at every opportunity. There were coast-to-coast keynote addresses, books to be written, and lives to save. We even planned a full-length documentary. Frankly, the frenetic pace was unsustainable. Thankfully, with time comes a new sense of balance.

As we move forward through the year to come, my focus will be on fewer projects, allowing me to really go deep. Our new website will continue to grow as we add resources aimed at helping all affected by brain injury, I will stay the course as our social community continues to thrive, and of course, HOPE Magazine will continue to evolve for the better. We have chosen these specific ways to advocate for a simple reason – they allow more lives to be touched. Less will indeed be best.

We are now living in an age where global communities are a reality. Having the ability to be a resource for others living lives affected by brain injury of all kinds adds a sense of purpose to what many might deem a tragedy.

From Sarah and I to you and yours, our best wishes for health and happiness this New Year.

~David & Sarah